BREAST CANCER COOKBOOK

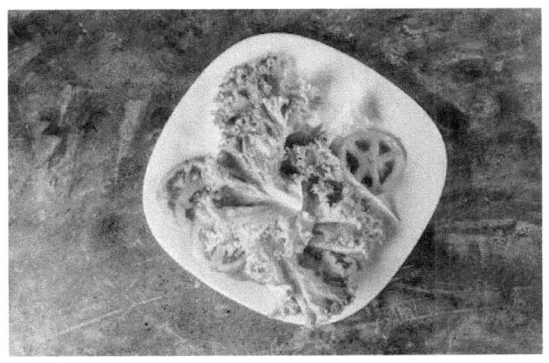

DR. JESSICA SMITH

Copyright © 2024 by DR. JESSICA SMITH

All rights reserved.

No part of this book may be reproduced, stored in a retrieval system, or transmitted, in any form or by any means, electronic, mechanical, photocopying, recording, or otherwise, without prior written permission from the publisher, except for brief quotations embodied in critical articles or reviews.

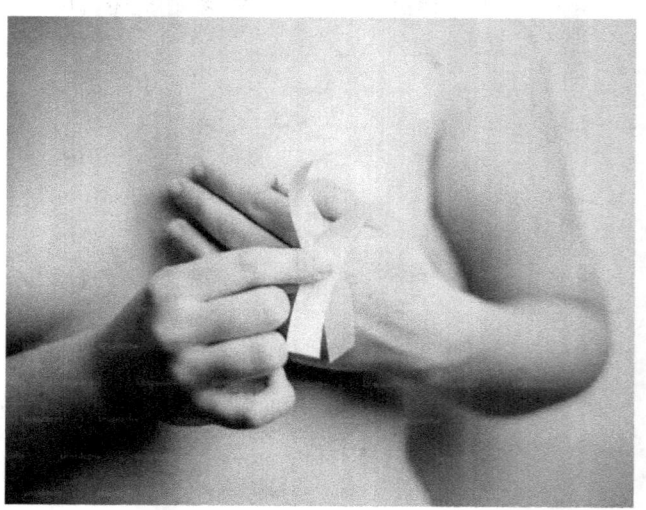

TABLE OF CONTENTS

CHAPTER ONE 7

How to Use this Cookbook. 7

Understanding Breast Cancer Cookbook 9

Benefits of Breast Cancer Cookbook 10

Guidelines for Breast Cancer Cookbook 12

Causes of Breast Cancer 14

Types of Breast Cancer 16

Symptoms of Breast Cancer 17

Risk Factor of Breast Cancer 18

CHAPTER TWO 21

Breast Cancer Breakfast Recipes 21

1: Berry Quinoa Breakfast Bowl 21

2: Avocado Toast with Smoked Salmon 23

3: Greek Yogurt Parfait with Granola and Berries. 24

4: Spinach and Feta Egg Muffins 26

5: Overnight Oats with Almond Butter and Banana 28

6: Veggie and Goat Cheese Frittata 29

7: Spinach and Mushroom Omelette 31

8: Blueberry Almond Smoothie 34

9: Chia Seed Pudding with Berries 36

10: Green Smoothie Bowl 38

Breast Cancer Lunch Recipes 39

1: Grilled Salmon Salad with Lemon-Dill Dressing 39

2: Quinoa Salad with Chickpeas and Avocado 41

3: Lentil and Vegetable Soup 44

4: Turkey and Avocado Wrap 46

5: Quinoa and Black Bean Stuffed Bell Peppers.... 48

6: Mediterranean Chickpea Salad 51

7: Mediterranean Tuna Salad 53

8: Veggie Quinoa Buddha Bowl 55

9: Spinach and Chickpea Salad with Lemon-Tahini Dressing 57

10: Turkey and Vegetable Stir-Fry 59

Breast Cancer Dinner Recipes 61

1: Baked Salmon with Asparagus and Lemon-Dill Sauce 61

2: Quinoa and Vegetable Stir-Fry 64

3: Baked Chicken Breast with Roasted Vegetables 66

4: Lentil and Vegetable Curry 69

5: Quinoa and Black Bean Stuffed Bell Peppers 71

6: Mediterranean Chickpea Salad 74

7: Turkey and Vegetable Skillet 76

8: Vegetable Lentil Soup 78

9: Lemon Garlic Shrimp with Quinoa and Broccoli 81

10: Mediterranean Stuffed Portobello Mushrooms 83

Breast Cancer Snacks Recipes 85

1: Greek Yogurt Parfait 85

2: Avocado Toast with Tomato and Basil 87

3: Hummus and Veggie Platter 89

4: Almond Butter Apple Slices 90

5: Berry and Nut Yogurt Parfait 92

6: Veggie Sushi Rolls 93

7: Edamame Hummus with Crudites 95

8: Almond Butter and Banana Rice Cakes 97

9: Cottage Cheese and Fruit Bowl 98

10: Spinach and Feta Stuffed Mushrooms 100

CONCLUSION 103

CHAPTER ONE

How to Use this Cookbook.

Read the Introduction: Start by reading the introduction of the cookbook. This section often provides valuable information about the relationship between nutrition and breast cancer, as well as tips for using the cookbook effectively.

Consult with Your Healthcare Provider: Before making any significant changes to your diet, it's essential to consult with your healthcare provider, especially if you're undergoing treatment for breast cancer.

Understand the Guidelines: Pay attention to any guidelines or recommendations provided in the cookbook regarding ingredients, portion sizes, and meal frequency.

Plan Your Meals: Take some time to plan your meals based on the recipes in the cookbook. Consider your schedule, preferences, and nutritional needs when making your meal plan.

Shop for Ingredients: Make a list of ingredients you'll need for the recipes you've chosen and head to the grocery store.

Try to stick to your list to avoid purchasing unnecessary items.

Prepare Your Kitchen: Before you start cooking, make sure your kitchen is equipped with all the necessary tools and utensils. Gather pots, pans, knives, cutting boards, and any other equipment you'll need.

Follow the Recipes: When cooking, carefully follow the recipes in the cookbook, paying attention to measurements, cooking times, and instructions. Feel free to get creative and make substitutions or modifications to suit your taste preferences.

Enjoy Your Meals: Once your meals are prepared, take the time to savor them. Eating mindfully can enhance your enjoyment of food and help you stay connected to your body's hunger and fullness cues.

Listen to Your Body: Pay attention to how your body responds to the meals you've prepared. Notice any changes in energy levels, digestion, or overall well-being. Adjust your diet as needed based on how you feel.

Understanding Breast Cancer Cookbook

Understanding this breast cancer cookbook involves recognizing its role as a resource tailored to the unique dietary needs and challenges faced by individuals impacted by breast cancer.

This cookbook typically offer a wealth of information beyond mere recipes. They often delve into the science behind nutrition and its impact on cancer prevention, treatment, and overall well-being.

Breast cancer cookbooks are designed to empower individuals with knowledge about the foods that can support their health journey.

They provide insights into ingredients known for their anti-inflammatory, antioxidant, and immune-boosting properties, all of which are crucial for combating the disease and supporting the body during treatment.

This cookbook often address common side effects of breast cancer treatment, such as fatigue, nausea, and changes in appetite or taste perception.

They offer practical tips and recipes specifically tailored to alleviate these symptoms, making mealtime more manageable and enjoyable.

It becomes a valuable tool not only for nourishing the body but also for fostering a sense of empowerment and control over one's health journey.

Benefits of Breast Cancer Cookbook

Breast cancer cookbooks offer a myriad of benefits to individuals navigating the complexities of a breast cancer diagnosis and treatment journey.

Firstly, they provide a sense of empowerment and control over one's health by offering practical guidance on nutrition tailored specifically to the needs of those affected by breast cancer.

This cookbook emphasize the importance of a balanced diet rich in nutrients that support the body's immune system, aid in recovery, and reduce the risk of cancer recurrence.

By incorporating recipes featuring ingredients known for their anti-inflammatory and antioxidant properties, such as fruits, vegetables, whole grains, and lean proteins, individuals can optimize their nutritional intake to support overall well-being.

Breast cancer cookbooks address common challenges experienced during treatment, such as loss of appetite, changes in taste perception, and digestive issues. They offer creative and flavorful recipes designed to alleviate these symptoms while ensuring adequate nourishment.

Beyond the kitchen, these cookbooks serve as a valuable educational resource, providing insights into the science behind nutrition and cancer, empowering individuals to make informed dietary choices.

They foster a sense of community and solidarity among those impacted by breast cancer, offering comfort, inspiration, and practical advice from others who have walked a similar path.

Breast cancer cookbooks are more than just collections of recipes; they are comprehensive guides to nurturing the body, supporting recovery, and promoting overall health and well-being throughout the breast cancer journey.

Guidelines for Breast Cancer Cookbook

Breast cancer cookbooks typically offer guidelines and recommendations to help individuals navigate their dietary choices during and after treatment.

These guidelines are designed to optimize nutrition, manage side effects, and support overall well-being. Here are some common guidelines found in breast cancer cookbooks:

Focus on Whole Foods: Emphasize whole, unprocessed foods such as fruits, vegetables, whole grains, lean proteins, and healthy fats. These foods provide essential nutrients and antioxidants that support the body's immune system and overall health.

Limit Processed Foods: Minimize intake of processed foods high in sugar, unhealthy fats, and additives, as these can contribute to inflammation and undermine health.

Stay Hydrated: Drink plenty of water throughout the day to stay hydrated, which is essential for overall health and well-being, especially during treatment.

Balance Macronutrients: Aim for a balanced diet that includes carbohydrates, proteins, and fats in appropriate proportions to support energy levels and overall health.

Manage Portions: Pay attention to portion sizes to prevent overeating and promote weight management, which is important for reducing the risk of cancer recurrence and maintaining overall health.

Adapt Recipes: Be flexible with recipes to accommodate individual preferences, dietary restrictions, and any side effects of treatment, such as changes in appetite or taste perception.

Seek Professional Guidance: Consult with a registered dietitian or healthcare provider for personalized dietary recommendations tailored to your specific needs and health goals.

Listen to Your Body: Pay attention to how your body responds to different foods and adjust your diet accordingly. Trust your instincts and eat intuitively to meet your nutritional needs.

Practice Mindful Eating: Practice mindfulness during meals by eating slowly, savoring each bite, and paying attention to hunger and fullness cues. This can help improve digestion and promote a healthy relationship with food.

Stay Informed: Stay informed about the latest research on nutrition and breast cancer, and be open to incorporating new dietary recommendations into your routine to support optimal health and well-being.

Causes of Breast Cancer

Breast cancer is a complex disease with multiple contributing factors, and its exact causes are not always clear.

However, researchers have identified several factors that may increase the risk of developing breast cancer:

Genetics: Inherited gene mutations, such as BRCA1 and BRCA2, significantly increase the risk of developing breast cancer.

These mutations are more common in certain populations and can be passed down from one generation to the next.

Family History: A family history of breast cancer, especially in close relatives like mother, sister, or daughter, can increase an individual's risk of developing the disease.

Age: The risk of breast cancer increases with age, with the majority of cases diagnosed in women over 50 years old. However, younger women can also develop breast cancer, albeit less frequently.

Hormonal Factors: Excessive exposure to estrogen over a lifetime, such as early onset of menstruation, late menopause, or hormone replacement therapy, can increase the risk of breast cancer.

Personal History: Women who have previously been diagnosed with breast cancer have a higher risk of developing a new cancer in the same breast or the other breast.

Lifestyle Factors: Certain lifestyle choices, such as excessive alcohol consumption, smoking, lack of physical activity, and poor diet, may contribute to an increased risk of breast cancer.

Environmental Exposures: Exposure to environmental toxins, radiation, and certain chemicals may increase the risk of developing breast cancer, although the extent of their contribution is still being studied.

Types of Breast Cancer

Breast cancer is not a single disease but rather a diverse group of cancers that originate in the breast tissue.

The specific type of breast cancer depends on where it begins in the breast, the presence of certain proteins, and other factors.

Here are some common types of breast cancer:

Ductal Carcinoma in Situ (DCIS): This is a non-invasive type of breast cancer where abnormal cells are found in the lining of the breast milk ducts. DCIS is considered an early stage of breast cancer and may or may not progress to invasive breast cancer if left untreated.

Invasive Ductal Carcinoma (IDC): IDC is the most common type of breast cancer, accounting for about 80% of all cases. It begins in the milk ducts of the breast and then invades nearby tissues in the breast.

Invasive Lobular Carcinoma (ILC): This type of breast cancer begins in the lobules, which are the glands that produce milk. ILC accounts for about 10-15% of all breast cancers.

Triple-Negative Breast Cancer: This is a subtype of breast cancer that lacks estrogen receptors, progesterone receptors, and HER2 protein. It tends to be more aggressive and less responsive to hormone therapy or targeted therapies.

HER2-Positive Breast Cancer: This type of breast cancer overexpresses the HER2 protein, which promotes the growth of cancer cells. HER2-positive breast cancer can be more aggressive but is often treated with targeted therapies that specifically inhibit the HER2 protein.

Symptoms of Breast Cancer

Breast cancer symptoms can vary widely among individuals, and some people may experience no symptoms at all, especially in the early stages of the disease.

Here are some common symptoms to watch for:

Lump or Mass: The most common symptom of breast cancer is a lump or mass in the breast tissue or underarm area. These lumps may feel firm, irregular in shape, and may or may not be painful.

Changes in Breast Size or Shape: Breast cancer can cause changes in breast size, shape, or contour.

One breast may become noticeably larger or smaller than the other, or the shape of the breast may change.

Changes in the Skin: Skin changes such as redness, swelling, dimpling, or puckering of the breast skin, resembling an orange peel, may indicate breast cancer.

Nipple Changes: Changes in the nipple, such as inversion (turning inward), discharge (other than breast milk), or scaling or crusting of the nipple or surrounding area, should be evaluated by a healthcare professional.

Breast Pain or Tenderness: While breast pain is more commonly associated with benign conditions, persistent or unusual breast pain or tenderness that does not resolve should be investigated further.

Changes in Breast Texture: Some women may notice changes in the texture of their breast tissue, such as thickening or hardening, which could be a sign of breast cancer.

Risk Factor of Breast Cancer

Breast cancer risk factors are diverse and multifaceted, encompassing a range of genetic, environmental, hormonal, and lifestyle factors. Understanding these risk factors can help individuals and healthcare professionals identify those at higher risk and implement appropriate preventive measures.

Here are some common risk factors associated with breast cancer:

Age: The risk of breast cancer increases with age, with the majority of cases diagnosed in women over 50 years old.

Gender: Although breast cancer can affect men, it is much more common in women, making female gender a significant risk factor.

Family History and Genetics: A family history of breast cancer, especially in first-degree relatives (mother, sister, daughter), and inherited genetic mutations such as BRCA1 and BRCA2 significantly increase the risk of developing breast cancer.

Personal History of Breast Cancer or Certain Non-Cancerous Breast Diseases: Women who have previously been diagnosed with breast cancer, ductal carcinoma in situ (DCIS), or lobular carcinoma in situ (LCIS) have a higher risk of developing breast cancer again.

Hormonal Factors: Early onset of menstruation (before age 12), late menopause (after age 55), hormone replacement therapy (HRT), and never having children or having the first child after age 30 can increase the risk of breast cancer due to prolonged exposure to estrogen.

Lifestyle Factors: Factors such as excessive alcohol consumption, smoking, lack of physical activity, obesity, and poor diet high in processed foods and saturated fats may increase the risk of breast cancer.

Radiation Exposure: Previous radiation therapy to the chest, such as for the treatment of Hodgkin lymphoma, increases the risk of developing breast cancer later in life.

Race and Ethnicity: While breast cancer can affect women of all races and ethnicities, some groups, such as Ashkenazi Jewish women, have a higher risk due to genetic factors.

Dense Breast Tissue: Women with dense breast tissue, as seen on mammograms, have a higher risk of breast cancer.

Exposure to Environmental Factors: Exposure to certain environmental toxins, chemicals, and pollutants may increase the risk of breast cancer, although the extent of their contribution is still being studied.

CHAPTER TWO

Breast Cancer Breakfast Recipes

1: Berry Quinoa Breakfast Bowl

Ingredients:

- 1/2 cup quinoa
- 1 cup water or almond milk
- 1/2 cup mixed berries (such as strawberries, blueberries, raspberries)
- 1 tablespoon honey or maple syrup
- 2 tablespoons chopped almonds or walnuts
- 1/2 teaspoon cinnamon
- Optional toppings: Greek yogurt, chia seeds, flaxseeds

Instructions:

- Rinse the quinoa under cold water.
- In a saucepan, combine quinoa and water (or almond milk) and bring to a boil.

- Reduce heat to low, cover, and simmer for 15 minutes or until quinoa is cooked and liquid is absorbed.
- In a serving bowl, mix cooked quinoa with berries, honey (or maple syrup), chopped nuts, and cinnamon.
- Serve warm, optionally topped with Greek yogurt, chia seeds, or flaxseeds for added protein and fiber.

Health Benefits:

- Quinoa is a whole grain rich in protein, fiber, and essential nutrients like iron and magnesium, which support overall health and well-being.
- Berries are packed with antioxidants, vitamins, and phytochemicals that help reduce inflammation and support immune function.
- Nuts provide healthy fats, protein, and micronutrients, contributing to heart health and satiety.

Preparation Time: Approximately 20 minutes.

2: Avocado Toast with Smoked Salmon

Ingredients:

- 2 slices whole grain bread
- 1 ripe avocado
- 4 ounces smoked salmon
- 1 tablespoon lemon juice
- Salt and pepper to taste
- Optional toppings: cherry tomatoes, microgreens, red onion slices

Instructions:

- Toast the slices of whole grain bread until golden brown.
- Mash the ripe avocado in a small bowl and mix with lemon juice, salt, and pepper.
- Spread the mashed avocado evenly onto each slice of toast.
- Top the avocado toast with slices of smoked salmon.
- Garnish with optional toppings like cherry tomatoes, microgreens, or red onion slices, if desired.

Health Benefits:

- Whole grain bread provides complex carbohydrates, fiber, and essential nutrients, supporting sustained energy levels and digestive health.
- Avocado is rich in heart-healthy monounsaturated fats, fiber, and vitamins, promoting satiety and overall cardiovascular health.
- Smoked salmon is a good source of protein, omega-3 fatty acids, and vitamin D, supporting muscle repair, brain function, and bone health.

Preparation Time: Approximately 10 minutes.

3: Greek Yogurt Parfait with Granola and Berries

Ingredients:

- 1 cup Greek yogurt (plain or flavored)
- 1/2 cup granola (choose low-sugar or homemade)
- 1/2 cup mixed berries (such as strawberries, blueberries, raspberries)
- 1 tablespoon honey or maple syrup (optional)

- 1 tablespoon chopped nuts (such as almonds, walnuts, or pecans)
- Optional toppings: shredded coconut, chia seeds, flaxseeds

Instructions:

- In a serving glass or bowl, layer Greek yogurt, granola, and mixed berries.
- Drizzle with honey or maple syrup if desired.
- Repeat the layers until the glass or bowl is filled.
- Top with chopped nuts and optional toppings like shredded coconut, chia seeds, or flaxseeds for added texture and nutrition.
- Serve immediately and enjoy!

Health Benefits:

- Greek yogurt is high in protein, calcium, and probiotics, which support digestive health and immune function.
- Granola provides complex carbohydrates, fiber, and essential nutrients, offering sustained energy and promoting satiety.

- Berries are rich in antioxidants, vitamins, and fiber, which help reduce inflammation and support overall health.

Preparation Time: Approximately 5 minutes.

4: Spinach and Feta Egg Muffins

Ingredients:

- 6 eggs
- 1 cup fresh spinach, chopped
- 1/2 cup crumbled feta cheese
- 1/4 cup diced tomatoes
- 1/4 cup diced bell peppers
- Salt and pepper to taste
- Cooking spray or olive oil for greasing muffin tin

Instructions:

- Preheat the oven to 350°F (175°C) and grease a muffin tin with cooking spray or olive oil.
- In a mixing bowl, whisk together eggs, salt, and pepper.

- Stir in chopped spinach, crumbled feta cheese, diced tomatoes, and diced bell peppers until well combined.
- Pour the egg mixture evenly into each muffin cup, filling each about 3/4 full.
- Bake in the preheated oven for 20-25 minutes or until the egg muffins are set and lightly golden on top.
- Allow the egg muffins to cool slightly before removing them from the muffin tin.
- Serve warm or refrigerate for later use.

Health Benefits:

- Eggs are a good source of high-quality protein, vitamins, and minerals, supporting muscle repair and overall health.
- Spinach is rich in iron, vitamins, and antioxidants, promoting heart health and immune function.
- Feta cheese adds flavor and provides calcium and protein, contributing to bone health and satiety.

Preparation Time: Approximately 30 minutes (including baking time).

5: Overnight Oats with Almond Butter and Banana

Ingredients:

- 1/2 cup rolled oats
- 1/2 cup almond milk (or any milk of choice)
- 1 tablespoon almond butter
- 1/2 ripe banana, mashed
- 1 tablespoon honey or maple syrup (optional)
- 1 tablespoon chia seeds
- Optional toppings: sliced banana, chopped nuts, cinnamon

Instructions:

- In a mason jar or airtight container, combine rolled oats, almond milk, almond butter, mashed banana, honey (or maple syrup), and chia seeds.
- Stir well to combine all ingredients.
- Cover the jar or container and refrigerate overnight or for at least 4 hours to allow the oats to soften and the flavors to meld.

- Before serving, give the oats a good stir and adjust the consistency with more almond milk if desired.
- Top with sliced banana, chopped nuts, and a sprinkle of cinnamon, if desired.
- Enjoy chilled straight from the fridge or warm it up in the microwave if preferred.

Health Benefits:

- Rolled oats are rich in fiber, providing sustained energy and supporting digestive health.
- Almond butter offers healthy fats, protein, and vitamin E, contributing to heart health and satiety.
- Bananas are a good source of potassium, vitamins, and natural sugars, providing a quick energy boost and aiding in muscle function.

Preparation Time: Approximately 5 minutes (plus chilling time).

6: Veggie and Goat Cheese Frittata

Ingredients:

- 6 eggs
- 1/2 cup diced bell peppers (any color)

- 1/2 cup diced zucchini
- 1/4 cup diced red onion
- 1/4 cup crumbled goat cheese
- 2 tablespoons chopped fresh parsley or basil
- Salt and pepper to taste
- Cooking spray or olive oil for greasing skillet

Instructions:

- Preheat the oven to 350°F (175°C).
- In a mixing bowl, whisk together eggs, salt, and pepper until well combined.
- Heat a skillet over medium heat and lightly grease with cooking spray or olive oil.
- Add diced bell peppers, zucchini, and red onion to the skillet and sauté for 3-4 minutes until vegetables are slightly softened.
- Pour the whisked eggs evenly over the sautéed vegetables in the skillet.
- Sprinkle crumbled goat cheese and chopped fresh herbs evenly over the eggs.

- Transfer the skillet to the preheated oven and bake for 15-20 minutes or until the frittata is set and lightly golden on top.
- Remove from the oven and let it cool slightly before slicing.
- Serve warm or at room temperature.

Health Benefits:

- Eggs provide high-quality protein, vitamins, and minerals, supporting muscle repair and overall health.
- Bell peppers and zucchini are rich in vitamins, minerals, and antioxidants, promoting immune function and heart health.
- Goat cheese adds flavor and provides calcium and protein, contributing to bone health and satiety.

Preparation Time: Approximately 30 minutes (including baking time).

7: Spinach and Mushroom Omelette

Ingredients:

- 2 large eggs

- 1/2 cup fresh spinach, chopped
- 1/4 cup sliced mushrooms
- 1/4 cup diced tomatoes
- 1/4 cup shredded low-fat cheese (such as mozzarella or cheddar)
- 1 tablespoon olive oil
- Salt and pepper to taste
- Optional toppings: salsa, avocado slices, chopped parsley

Instructions:

- In a small bowl, whisk the eggs until well beaten. Season with salt and pepper.
- Heat olive oil in a non-stick skillet over medium heat.
- Add the chopped spinach, sliced mushrooms, and diced tomatoes to the skillet. Cook for 2-3 minutes until vegetables are softened.
- Pour the beaten eggs over the cooked vegetables in the skillet. Allow the eggs to cook undisturbed for a minute.

- Using a spatula, gently lift the edges of the omelette and tilt the skillet to let the uncooked eggs flow to the bottom.
- Once the omelette is mostly set but still slightly runny on top, sprinkle shredded cheese evenly over one side of the omelette.
- Carefully fold the other side of the omelette over the cheese to create a half-moon shape.
- Cook for another 1-2 minutes until the cheese is melted and the omelette is cooked through.
- Slide the omelette onto a plate and garnish with optional toppings like salsa, avocado slices, or chopped parsley.
- Serve hot and enjoy!

Health Benefits:

- Eggs are rich in high-quality protein and essential nutrients, supporting muscle repair and overall health.
- Spinach and mushrooms provide vitamins, minerals, and antioxidants, promoting immune function and heart health.

- Low-fat cheese adds flavor and protein, contributing to bone health and satiety.

Preparation Time: Approximately 15 minutes.

8: Blueberry Almond Smoothie

Ingredients:

- 1/2 cup frozen blueberries
- 1 ripe banana
- 1/4 cup plain Greek yogurt
- 1 tablespoon almond butter
- 1/2 cup almond milk (or any milk of choice)
- 1 tablespoon honey or maple syrup (optional)
- Optional add-ins: spinach, chia seeds, flaxseeds, protein powder

Instructions:

- Combine frozen blueberries, ripe banana, Greek yogurt, almond butter, almond milk, and honey (or maple syrup) in a blender.
- Blend on high until smooth and creamy. If the smoothie is too thick, add more almond milk as needed to reach the desired consistency.

- Taste and adjust sweetness if necessary by adding more honey or maple syrup.
- For added nutrition, consider adding optional add-ins like spinach (for extra greens), chia seeds or flaxseeds (for omega-3 fatty acids and fiber), or protein powder (for additional protein).
- Blend again until all ingredients are well combined.
- Pour the smoothie into a glass and serve immediately.
- Enjoy as a nutritious and refreshing breakfast option!

Health Benefits:

- Blueberries are rich in antioxidants, vitamins, and fiber, promoting brain health and reducing inflammation.
- Bananas provide natural sugars, potassium, and vitamins, offering a quick energy boost and supporting muscle function.
- Almond butter adds healthy fats, protein, and vitamin E, contributing to heart health and satiety.

Preparation Time: Approximately 5 minutes.

9: Chia Seed Pudding with Berries

Ingredients:

- 1/4 cup chia seeds
- 1 cup almond milk (or any milk of choice)
- 1 tablespoon honey or maple syrup
- 1/2 teaspoon vanilla extract
- 1/2 cup mixed berries (such as strawberries, blueberries, raspberries)
- Optional toppings: sliced almonds, shredded coconut, additional berries

Instructions:

- In a bowl or mason jar, combine chia seeds, almond milk, honey (or maple syrup), and vanilla extract. Stir well to combine.
- Cover the bowl or jar and refrigerate for at least 2 hours or overnight to allow the chia seeds to absorb the liquid and thicken into a pudding-like consistency.
- Stir the chia seed pudding mixture well before serving to ensure an even texture.

- Divide the chia seed pudding into serving bowls or glasses.
- Top with mixed berries and any optional toppings such as sliced almonds, shredded coconut, or additional berries.
- Serve chilled and enjoy!

Health Benefits:

- Chia seeds are rich in fiber, omega-3 fatty acids, and antioxidants, promoting digestive health, heart health, and reducing inflammation.
- Almond milk is a dairy-free alternative rich in calcium, vitamin E, and healthy fats, contributing to bone health and overall well-being.
- Berries are packed with vitamins, minerals, and antioxidants, supporting immune function, brain health, and reducing the risk of chronic diseases.

Preparation Time: Approximately 5 minutes (plus chilling time).

10: Green Smoothie Bowl

Ingredients:

- 1 ripe banana, frozen
- 1/2 cup frozen mango chunks
- 1 cup fresh spinach or kale leaves
- 1/2 cup almond milk (or any milk of choice)
- 1 tablespoon almond butter
- Optional toppings: sliced banana, granola, chia seeds, hemp seeds

Instructions:

- In a blender, combine frozen banana, frozen mango chunks, fresh spinach or kale leaves, almond milk, and almond butter.
- Blend on high until smooth and creamy, adding more almond milk if needed to reach the desired consistency.
- Pour the green smoothie into a bowl.
- Top with sliced banana, granola, chia seeds, hemp seeds, or any other desired toppings.
- Serve immediately and enjoy!

Health Benefits:

- Leafy greens like spinach and kale are rich in vitamins, minerals, and antioxidants, supporting immune function, bone health, and reducing inflammation.
- Bananas and mangoes provide natural sugars, vitamins, and minerals, offering a quick energy boost and aiding digestion.
- Almond butter adds healthy fats, protein, and vitamin E, contributing to heart health and satiety.

Preparation Time: Approximately 5 minutes.

Breast Cancer Lunch Recipes

1: Grilled Salmon Salad with Lemon-Dill Dressing

Ingredients:

- 2 salmon fillets
- 4 cups mixed salad greens (such as spinach, arugula, and romaine)
- 1 cucumber, sliced
- 1 cup cherry tomatoes, halved

- 1/4 red onion, thinly sliced
- 1/4 cup sliced almonds
- 2 tablespoons chopped fresh dill
- 1 lemon
- 2 tablespoons olive oil
- Salt and pepper to taste

Instructions:

- Preheat the grill to medium-high heat.
- Season the salmon fillets with salt, pepper, and a squeeze of lemon juice.
- Grill the salmon fillets for 4-5 minutes per side, or until cooked through and slightly charred. Remove from the grill and let them rest for a few minutes.
- In a large mixing bowl, combine the mixed salad greens, sliced cucumber, halved cherry tomatoes, thinly sliced red onion, and sliced almonds.
- In a small bowl, whisk together the juice of one lemon, olive oil, chopped fresh dill, salt, and pepper to make the dressing.
- Pour the lemon-dill dressing over the salad and toss until well combined.

- Divide the salad onto plates and top each serving with a grilled salmon fillet.
- Garnish with additional lemon wedges and fresh dill, if desired.
- Serve immediately and enjoy!

Health Benefits:

- Salmon is rich in omega-3 fatty acids, protein, and vitamin D, supporting heart health, brain function, and reducing inflammation.
- Leafy greens like spinach and arugula are packed with vitamins, minerals, and antioxidants, promoting immune function and reducing the risk of chronic diseases.
- Cucumbers and tomatoes provide hydration, vitamins, and antioxidants, supporting skin health and reducing inflammation.

Preparation Time: Approximately 20 minutes.

2: Quinoa Salad with Chickpeas and Avocado

Ingredients:

- 1 cup quinoa, rinsed

- 2 cups water or vegetable broth
- 1 can (15 ounces) chickpeas, drained and rinsed
- 1 red bell pepper, diced
- 1/2 cucumber, diced
- 1 avocado, diced
- 1/4 cup chopped fresh parsley
- 1/4 cup crumbled feta cheese (optional)
- Juice of 1 lemon
- 2 tablespoons olive oil
- Salt and pepper to taste

Instructions:

- In a medium saucepan, combine the rinsed quinoa and water or vegetable broth. Bring to a boil, then reduce heat to low, cover, and simmer for 15 minutes or until the quinoa is cooked and the liquid is absorbed.
- Once cooked, fluff the quinoa with a fork and let it cool to room temperature.
- In a large mixing bowl, combine the cooked quinoa, drained and rinsed chickpeas, diced red bell pepper,

- diced cucumber, diced avocado, and chopped fresh parsley.
- In a small bowl, whisk together the lemon juice, olive oil, salt, and pepper to make the dressing.
- Pour the dressing over the quinoa salad and toss until well combined.
- If desired, sprinkle crumbled feta cheese over the salad before serving.
- Serve chilled or at room temperature.
- Enjoy as a nutritious and satisfying lunch option!

Health Benefits:

- Quinoa is a gluten-free whole grain rich in protein, fiber, and essential nutrients, supporting digestive health and providing sustained energy.
- Chickpeas are a good source of plant-based protein, fiber, and vitamins, promoting heart health, stabilizing blood sugar levels, and reducing inflammation.
- Avocado provides healthy fats, vitamins, and minerals, supporting heart health, satiety, and reducing inflammation.

Preparation Time: Approximately 25 minutes.

3: Lentil and Vegetable Soup

Ingredients:

- 1 cup dried green or brown lentils, rinsed
- 4 cups vegetable broth
- 1 onion, diced
- 2 carrots, diced
- 2 celery stalks, diced
- 2 cloves garlic, minced
- 1 teaspoon ground cumin
- 1 teaspoon ground turmeric
- 1/2 teaspoon ground coriander
- 1/4 teaspoon red pepper flakes (optional)
- Salt and pepper to taste
- 2 tablespoons olive oil
- 2 tablespoons chopped fresh parsley or cilantro
- Lemon wedges for serving

Instructions:

- In a large pot, heat olive oil over medium heat. Add diced onion, carrots, and celery. Cook until softened, about 5 minutes.
- Add minced garlic, ground cumin, ground turmeric, ground coriander, and red pepper flakes (if using). Cook for another 1-2 minutes until fragrant.
- Add rinsed lentils and vegetable broth to the pot. Bring to a boil, then reduce heat to low and simmer, covered, for about 20-25 minutes or until lentils are tender.
- Season the soup with salt and pepper to taste. Adjust seasoning as needed.
- Serve the lentil and vegetable soup hot, garnished with chopped fresh parsley or cilantro, and lemon wedges on the side for squeezing over the soup.
- Enjoy as a comforting and nutritious lunch option!

Health Benefits:

- Lentils are a good source of plant-based protein, fiber, and vitamins, promoting heart health,

stabilizing blood sugar levels, and supporting digestive health.
- Vegetables like onions, carrots, and celery provide vitamins, minerals, and antioxidants, supporting immune function, reducing inflammation, and promoting overall health.
- Spices such as cumin, turmeric, and coriander add flavor and offer anti-inflammatory and antioxidant properties.

Preparation Time: Approximately 30 minutes.

4: Turkey and Avocado Wrap

Ingredients:

- 2 whole grain or gluten-free wraps
- 8 ounces cooked turkey breast, sliced
- 1 avocado, sliced
- 1 cup mixed salad greens (such as spinach, arugula, and romaine)
- 1/2 cup cherry tomatoes, halved
- 1/4 cup shredded carrots
- 1/4 cup hummus
- 2 tablespoons Greek yogurt (optional)

- Salt and pepper to taste

Instructions:

- Lay out the wraps on a clean work surface.
- Spread a layer of hummus onto each wrap, leaving a small border around the edges.
- Arrange sliced turkey breast, avocado slices, mixed salad greens, halved cherry tomatoes, and shredded carrots evenly over the hummus layer on each wrap.
- If desired, drizzle Greek yogurt over the fillings for added creaminess.
- Season with salt and pepper to taste.
- Roll up the wraps tightly, tucking in the sides as you go.
- Cut each wrap in half diagonally to serve, if desired.
- Serve immediately or wrap tightly in foil or parchment paper for later enjoyment.
- Enjoy as a delicious and satisfying lunch option!

Health Benefits:

- Whole grain wraps provide complex carbohydrates, fiber, and essential nutrients, promoting digestive health and providing sustained energy.
- Turkey breast is lean protein, low in saturated fat, and rich in vitamins and minerals, supporting muscle repair and overall health.
- Avocado offers healthy fats, vitamins, and minerals, promoting heart health, satiety, and reducing inflammation.

Preparation Time: Approximately 15 minutes.

5: Quinoa and Black Bean Stuffed Bell Peppers

Ingredients:

- 4 large bell peppers (any color), halved and seeds removed
- 1 cup cooked quinoa
- 1 can (15 ounces) black beans, drained and rinsed
- 1 cup corn kernels (fresh, frozen, or canned)
- 1/2 cup diced tomatoes

- 1/4 cup diced red onion
- 1/4 cup chopped fresh cilantro
- 1 teaspoon ground cumin
- 1/2 teaspoon chili powder
- Salt and pepper to taste
- 1/2 cup shredded cheese (such as cheddar or Monterey Jack), optional
- Sliced avocado and lime wedges for serving

Instructions:

- Preheat the oven to 375°F (190°C). Line a baking dish with parchment paper or lightly grease with olive oil.
- In a large mixing bowl, combine cooked quinoa, black beans, corn kernels, diced tomatoes, diced red onion, chopped fresh cilantro, ground cumin, chili powder, salt, and pepper. Stir well to combine.
- Arrange the halved bell peppers in the prepared baking dish, cut side up.
- Spoon the quinoa and black bean mixture evenly into each bell pepper half, pressing down gently to pack the filling.

- If using, sprinkle shredded cheese over the stuffed bell peppers.
- Cover the baking dish with foil and bake in the preheated oven for 25-30 minutes, or until the bell peppers are tender and the filling is heated through.
- Remove the foil and bake for an additional 5 minutes, or until the cheese is melted and bubbly.
- Remove from the oven and let cool slightly before serving.
- Serve the stuffed bell peppers hot, garnished with sliced avocado and lime wedges on the side for squeezing over the peppers.
- Enjoy as a flavorful and nutritious lunch option!

Health Benefits:

- Bell peppers are rich in vitamins, minerals, and antioxidants, supporting immune function, reducing inflammation, and promoting overall health.
- Quinoa is a gluten-free whole grain rich in protein, fiber, and essential nutrients, supporting digestive health and providing sustained energy.

- Black beans provide plant-based protein, fiber, vitamins, and minerals, promoting heart health, stabilizing blood sugar levels, and supporting digestive health.

Preparation Time: Approximately 45 minutes.

6: Mediterranean Chickpea Salad

Ingredients:

- 2 cans (15 ounces each) chickpeas, drained and rinsed
- 1 cup cherry tomatoes, halved
- 1 cucumber, diced
- 1/4 cup diced red onion
- 1/4 cup chopped fresh parsley
- 1/4 cup chopped fresh mint
- 1/4 cup crumbled feta cheese (optional)
- Juice of 1 lemon
- 2 tablespoons extra virgin olive oil
- 1 teaspoon dried oregano
- Salt and pepper to taste

Instructions:

- In a large mixing bowl, combine chickpeas, halved cherry tomatoes, diced cucumber, diced red onion, chopped fresh parsley, and chopped fresh mint.
- In a small bowl, whisk together the lemon juice, extra virgin olive oil, dried oregano, salt, and pepper to make the dressing.
- Pour the dressing over the chickpea salad and toss until well combined.
- If using, sprinkle crumbled feta cheese over the salad and toss gently to distribute.
- Taste and adjust seasoning as needed.
- Serve the Mediterranean chickpea salad chilled or at room temperature.
- Enjoy as a refreshing and nutritious lunch option!

Health Benefits:

- Chickpeas are a good source of plant-based protein, fiber, vitamins, and minerals, promoting heart health, stabilizing blood sugar levels, and supporting digestive health.

- Cherry tomatoes and cucumbers provide hydration, vitamins, minerals, and antioxidants, supporting immune function, reducing inflammation, and promoting overall health.
- Fresh herbs like parsley and mint add flavor and offer vitamins, minerals, and antioxidants.

Preparation Time: Approximately 15 minutes.

7: Mediterranean Tuna Salad

Ingredients:

- 2 cans (5 ounces each) tuna in water, drained
- 1/2 cup cherry tomatoes, halved
- 1/2 cucumber, diced
- 1/4 cup sliced Kalamata olives
- 1/4 cup diced red onion
- 2 tablespoons chopped fresh parsley
- 2 tablespoons extra virgin olive oil
- Juice of 1 lemon
- 1 teaspoon dried oregano
- Salt and pepper to taste
- Mixed salad greens for serving

Instructions:

- In a large mixing bowl, flake the drained tuna with a fork.
- Add halved cherry tomatoes, diced cucumber, sliced Kalamata olives, diced red onion, and chopped fresh parsley to the bowl with the tuna.
- In a small bowl, whisk together the extra virgin olive oil, lemon juice, dried oregano, salt, and pepper to make the dressing.
- Pour the dressing over the tuna salad mixture and toss until well combined.
- Taste and adjust seasoning as needed.
- Serve the Mediterranean tuna salad over a bed of mixed salad greens.
- Enjoy as a flavorful and satisfying lunch option!

Health Benefits:

- Tuna is rich in protein, omega-3 fatty acids, and vitamins, supporting muscle repair, brain function, and reducing inflammation.
- Cherry tomatoes, cucumbers, and red onions provide vitamins, minerals, and antioxidants, supporting

immune function, reducing inflammation, and promoting overall health.
- Olives and extra virgin olive oil offer healthy fats, antioxidants, and anti-inflammatory properties, supporting heart health and satiety.

Preparation Time: Approximately 15 minutes.

8: Veggie Quinoa Buddha Bowl

Ingredients:

- 1 cup cooked quinoa
- 1 cup roasted vegetables (such as sweet potatoes, broccoli, bell peppers)
- 1/2 cup cooked chickpeas
- 1/2 avocado, sliced
- 2 tablespoons hummus
- 1 tablespoon tahini
- Juice of 1 lemon
- Salt and pepper to taste
- Sprouts or microgreens for garnish (optional)

Instructions:

- In a serving bowl, arrange cooked quinoa, roasted vegetables, cooked chickpeas, and sliced avocado in separate sections.
- In a small bowl, whisk together hummus, tahini, lemon juice, salt, and pepper to make the dressing.
- Drizzle the dressing over the ingredients in the bowl.
- Garnish with sprouts or microgreens, if desired.
- Serve the veggie quinoa Buddha bowl immediately.
- Enjoy as a nourishing and satisfying lunch option!

Health Benefits:

- Quinoa is a gluten-free whole grain rich in protein, fiber, and essential nutrients, supporting digestive health and providing sustained energy.
- Roasted vegetables and chickpeas provide vitamins, minerals, and antioxidants, supporting immune function, reducing inflammation, and promoting overall health.
- Avocado offers healthy fats, vitamins, and minerals, promoting heart health, satiety, and reducing inflammation.

Preparation Time: Approximately 30 minutes (depending on roasting time for vegetables).

9: Spinach and Chickpea Salad with Lemon-Tahini Dressing

Ingredients:

- 4 cups baby spinach leaves
- 1 can (15 ounces) chickpeas, drained and rinsed
- 1/2 cup sliced cucumber
- 1/2 cup halved cherry tomatoes
- 1/4 cup sliced red onion
- 1/4 cup chopped fresh parsley
- 2 tablespoons tahini
- Juice of 1 lemon
- 2 tablespoons water
- 1 clove garlic, minced
- Salt and pepper to taste
- Optional toppings: toasted pine nuts, crumbled feta cheese

Instructions:

- In a large mixing bowl, combine baby spinach leaves, chickpeas, sliced cucumber, halved cherry tomatoes, sliced red onion, and chopped fresh parsley.
- In a small bowl, whisk together tahini, lemon juice, water, minced garlic, salt, and pepper to make the dressing. Adjust the consistency with more water if needed.
- Pour the dressing over the spinach and chickpea salad mixture. Toss until well coated.
- Taste and adjust seasoning as needed.
- Divide the salad into serving bowls.
- If desired, sprinkle toasted pine nuts and crumbled feta cheese over each serving.
- Serve immediately and enjoy!

Health Benefits:

- Spinach is rich in vitamins, minerals, and antioxidants, promoting immune function, bone health, and reducing inflammation.

- Chickpeas provide plant-based protein, fiber, vitamins, and minerals, supporting heart health, stabilizing blood sugar levels, and aiding digestion.
- Tahini offers healthy fats, protein, and minerals, promoting heart health, satiety, and reducing inflammation.

Preparation Time: Approximately 15 minutes.

10: Turkey and Vegetable Stir-Fry

Ingredients:

- 1 tablespoon olive oil
- 1 pound turkey breast, thinly sliced
- 2 cups mixed vegetables (such as bell peppers, broccoli, snap peas)
- 1/4 cup low-sodium soy sauce or tamari
- 2 tablespoons rice vinegar
- 1 tablespoon honey or maple syrup
- 2 cloves garlic, minced
- 1 teaspoon grated ginger
- 2 cups cooked brown rice or quinoa
- Sesame seeds for garnish (optional)
- Sliced green onions for garnish (optional)

Instructions:

- Heat olive oil in a large skillet or wok over medium-high heat.
- Add thinly sliced turkey breast to the skillet and cook until browned and cooked through, about 5-7 minutes. Remove from the skillet and set aside.
- In the same skillet, add mixed vegetables and stir-fry until tender-crisp, about 3-5 minutes.
- In a small bowl, whisk together low-sodium soy sauce or tamari, rice vinegar, honey or maple syrup, minced garlic, and grated ginger to make the sauce.
- Return the cooked turkey breast to the skillet with the vegetables.
- Pour the sauce over the turkey and vegetables. Stir to coat evenly and cook for an additional 2-3 minutes, until heated through.
- Serve the turkey and vegetable stir-fry over cooked brown rice or quinoa.
- Garnish with sesame seeds and sliced green onions, if desired.
- Enjoy hot as a flavorful and nutritious lunch option!

Health Benefits:

- Turkey breast is lean protein, low in saturated fat, and rich in vitamins and minerals, supporting muscle repair and overall health.
- Mixed vegetables provide vitamins, minerals, and antioxidants, supporting immune function, reducing inflammation, and promoting overall health.
- Brown rice or quinoa offer complex carbohydrates, fiber, and essential nutrients, supporting digestive health and providing sustained energy.

Preparation Time: Approximately 20 minutes.

Breast Cancer Dinner Recipes

1: Baked Salmon with Asparagus and Lemon-Dill Sauce

Ingredients:

- 4 salmon fillets
- 1 bunch asparagus, trimmed
- 2 tablespoons olive oil
- Salt and pepper to taste
- 1 lemon, sliced

- Fresh dill for garnish

For the Lemon-Dill Sauce:

- 1/4 cup plain Greek yogurt
- 1 tablespoon chopped fresh dill
- Juice of 1 lemon
- 1 teaspoon honey or maple syrup
- Salt and pepper to taste

Instructions:

- Preheat the oven to 400°F (200°C).
- Place the asparagus on a baking sheet and drizzle with olive oil. Season with salt and pepper, then toss to coat evenly.
- Arrange the asparagus in a single layer on one side of the baking sheet.
- Place the salmon fillets on the other side of the baking sheet. Drizzle with olive oil and season with salt and pepper.
- Place lemon slices on top of the salmon fillets.

- Bake in the preheated oven for 12-15 minutes, or until the salmon is cooked through and the asparagus is tender.
- While the salmon and asparagus are baking, prepare the lemon-dill sauce. In a small bowl, mix together Greek yogurt, chopped fresh dill, lemon juice, honey or maple syrup, salt, and pepper.
- Once the salmon and asparagus are cooked, remove from the oven.
- Serve the baked salmon and asparagus hot, garnished with fresh dill and accompanied by the lemon-dill sauce.
- Enjoy this delicious and nutritious dinner!

Health Benefits:

- Salmon is rich in omega-3 fatty acids, which have anti-inflammatory properties and may help reduce the risk of breast cancer recurrence.
- Asparagus is a good source of folate, vitamins A, C, and K, and antioxidants, which can help protect against cell damage and support immune health.

- Greek yogurt provides probiotics that support gut health and immune function, while also being a good source of protein and calcium.

Preparation Time: Approximately 20 minutes.

2: Quinoa and Vegetable Stir-Fry

Ingredients:

- 1 cup quinoa
- 2 cups water or vegetable broth
- 2 tablespoons olive oil
- 2 cloves garlic, minced
- 1 bell pepper, sliced
- 1 zucchini, sliced
- 1 cup broccoli florets
- 1 cup sliced mushrooms
- 1 carrot, sliced
- 1/4 cup soy sauce or tamari
- 2 tablespoons rice vinegar
- 1 tablespoon honey or maple syrup
- 1 teaspoon grated ginger
- Sesame seeds for garnish (optional)

- Sliced green onions for garnish (optional)

Instructions:

- Rinse the quinoa under cold water using a fine-mesh sieve. In a saucepan, combine the quinoa and water or vegetable broth. Bring to a boil, then reduce the heat to low, cover, and simmer for 15-20 minutes, or until the quinoa is cooked and the liquid is absorbed.
- While the quinoa is cooking, heat olive oil in a large skillet or wok over medium-high heat. Add minced garlic and sauté for 1 minute, until fragrant.
- Add sliced bell pepper, zucchini, broccoli florets, mushrooms, and carrot to the skillet. Stir-fry for 5-7 minutes, or until the vegetables are tender-crisp.
- In a small bowl, whisk together soy sauce or tamari, rice vinegar, honey or maple syrup, and grated ginger to make the sauce.
- Add the cooked quinoa to the skillet with the stir-fried vegetables. Pour the sauce over the quinoa and vegetables. Stir to coat evenly and cook for an additional 2-3 minutes, until heated through.

- Serve the quinoa and vegetable stir-fry hot, garnished with sesame seeds and sliced green onions, if desired.
- Enjoy this flavorful and nutritious dinner!

Health Benefits:

- Quinoa is a gluten-free whole grain rich in protein, fiber, and essential nutrients, which can help support digestion and provide long-lasting energy.
- Vegetables such as bell peppers, zucchini, broccoli, mushrooms, and carrots are rich in vitamins, minerals, and antioxidants, which can help reduce inflammation and support overall health.
- Garlic and ginger provide additional flavor and contain compounds that may have anticancer properties.

Preparation Time: Approximately 30 minutes.

3: Baked Chicken Breast with Roasted Vegetables

Ingredients:

- 4 boneless, skinless chicken breasts
- 2 tablespoons olive oil

- 2 teaspoons dried Italian seasoning
- Salt and pepper to taste
- 1 pound mixed vegetables (such as bell peppers, zucchini, cherry tomatoes, red onion)
- 2 tablespoons balsamic vinegar
- 2 cloves garlic, minced
- Fresh basil leaves for garnish (optional)

Instructions:

- Preheat the oven to 400°F (200°C).
- Place the chicken breasts on a baking sheet lined with parchment paper or aluminum foil.
- Drizzle olive oil over the chicken breasts and sprinkle with dried Italian seasoning, salt, and pepper. Rub the seasoning evenly over the chicken.
- In a mixing bowl, toss the mixed vegetables with olive oil, balsamic vinegar, minced garlic, salt, and pepper.
- Arrange the vegetables around the chicken breasts on the baking sheet.

- Bake in the preheated oven for 20-25 minutes, or until the chicken is cooked through and the vegetables are tender.
- Once cooked, remove from the oven and let the chicken rest for a few minutes before serving.
- Garnish with fresh basil leaves, if desired.
- Serve the baked chicken breast with roasted vegetables hot.
- Enjoy this wholesome and flavorful dinner!

Health Benefits:

- Chicken breast is a lean source of protein, which is essential for muscle repair and immune function.
- Mixed vegetables provide vitamins, minerals, and antioxidants, which can help reduce inflammation and support overall health.
- Olive oil and balsamic vinegar offer healthy fats and flavor without adding excessive calories, and garlic adds additional flavor and potential health benefits.

Preparation Time: Approximately 30 minutes.

4: Lentil and Vegetable Curry

Ingredients:

- 1 cup dried green or brown lentils, rinsed
- 4 cups vegetable broth
- 2 tablespoons olive oil
- 1 onion, diced
- 2 cloves garlic, minced
- 1 tablespoon grated ginger
- 2 carrots, diced
- 1 bell pepper, diced
- 1 zucchini, diced
- 1 cup canned diced tomatoes
- 2 tablespoons curry powder
- 1 teaspoon ground cumin
- 1 teaspoon ground turmeric
- Salt and pepper to taste
- 1/4 cup chopped fresh cilantro for garnish
- Cooked brown rice or quinoa for serving

Instructions:

- In a large pot, heat olive oil over medium heat. Add diced onion and sauté until translucent, about 5 minutes.
- Add minced garlic and grated ginger to the pot. Sauté for another 1-2 minutes until fragrant.
- Add diced carrots, bell pepper, and zucchini to the pot. Cook for 5 minutes, stirring occasionally.
- Stir in curry powder, ground cumin, ground turmeric, salt, and pepper. Cook for 1 minute until the spices are fragrant.
- Add rinsed lentils, vegetable broth, and canned diced tomatoes to the pot. Bring to a boil, then reduce heat to low and simmer, covered, for 20-25 minutes or until the lentils are tender.
- Once cooked, taste and adjust seasoning as needed.
- Serve the lentil and vegetable curry hot, garnished with chopped fresh cilantro.
- Enjoy with cooked brown rice or quinoa for a complete and satisfying meal!

Health Benefits:

- Lentils are a good source of plant-based protein, fiber, vitamins, and minerals, which can help support digestion and provide sustained energy.
- Vegetables such as carrots, bell peppers, and zucchini are rich in vitamins, minerals, and antioxidants, which can help reduce inflammation and support overall health.
- Spices like curry powder, cumin, and turmeric not only add flavor but also offer potential health benefits, including anti-inflammatory and antioxidant properties.

Preparation Time: Approximately 45 minutes.

5: Quinoa and Black Bean Stuffed Bell Peppers

Ingredients:

- 4 large bell peppers (any color), halved and seeds removed
- 1 cup cooked quinoa
- 1 can (15 ounces) black beans, drained and rinsed

- 1 cup corn kernels (fresh, frozen, or canned)
- 1/2 cup diced tomatoes
- 1/4 cup diced red onion
- 1/4 cup chopped fresh cilantro
- 1 teaspoon ground cumin
- 1/2 teaspoon chili powder
- Salt and pepper to taste
- 1/2 cup shredded cheese (such as cheddar or Monterey Jack), optional
- Sliced avocado and lime wedges for serving

Instructions:

- Preheat the oven to 375°F (190°C). Line a baking dish with parchment paper or lightly grease with olive oil.
- In a large mixing bowl, combine cooked quinoa, black beans, corn kernels, diced tomatoes, diced red onion, chopped fresh cilantro, ground cumin, chili powder, salt, and pepper. Stir well to combine.
- Arrange the halved bell peppers in the prepared baking dish, cut side up.

- Spoon the quinoa and black bean mixture evenly into each bell pepper half, pressing down gently to pack the filling.
- If using, sprinkle shredded cheese over the stuffed bell peppers.
- Cover the baking dish with foil and bake in the preheated oven for 25-30 minutes, or until the bell peppers are tender and the filling is heated through.
- Remove the foil and bake for an additional 5 minutes, or until the cheese is melted and bubbly.
- Remove from the oven and let cool slightly before serving.
- Serve the stuffed bell peppers hot, garnished with sliced avocado and lime wedges on the side for squeezing over the peppers.
- Enjoy as a flavorful and nutritious dinner option!

Health Benefits:

- Bell peppers are rich in vitamins, minerals, and antioxidants, supporting immune function, reducing inflammation, and promoting overall health.

- Quinoa is a gluten-free whole grain rich in protein, fiber, and essential nutrients, supporting digestive health and providing sustained energy.
- Black beans provide plant-based protein, fiber, vitamins, and minerals, promoting heart health, stabilizing blood sugar levels, and supporting digestive health.

Preparation Time: Approximately 45 minutes.

6: Mediterranean Chickpea Salad

Ingredients:

- 2 cans (15 ounces each) chickpeas, drained and rinsed
- 1 cup cherry tomatoes, halved
- 1 cucumber, diced
- 1/4 cup diced red onion
- 1/4 cup chopped fresh parsley
- 1/4 cup chopped fresh mint
- 1/4 cup crumbled feta cheese (optional)
- Juice of 1 lemon
- 2 tablespoons extra virgin olive oil
- 1 teaspoon dried oregano

- Salt and pepper to taste

Instructions:

- In a large mixing bowl, combine chickpeas, halved cherry tomatoes, diced cucumber, diced red onion, chopped fresh parsley, and chopped fresh mint.
- In a small bowl, whisk together the lemon juice, extra virgin olive oil, dried oregano, salt, and pepper to make the dressing.
- Pour the dressing over the chickpea salad and toss until well combined.
- If using, sprinkle crumbled feta cheese over the salad and toss gently to distribute.
- Taste and adjust seasoning as needed.
- Serve the Mediterranean chickpea salad chilled or at room temperature.
- Enjoy as a refreshing and nutritious dinner option!

Health Benefits:

- Chickpeas are a good source of plant-based protein, fiber, vitamins, and minerals, promoting heart health, stabilizing blood sugar levels, and supporting digestive health.

- Cherry tomatoes and cucumbers provide hydration, vitamins, minerals, and antioxidants, supporting immune function, reducing inflammation, and promoting overall health.
- Fresh herbs like parsley and mint add flavor and offer vitamins, minerals, and antioxidants.

Preparation Time: Approximately 15 minutes.

7: Turkey and Vegetable Skillet

Ingredients:

- 1 pound lean ground turkey
- 1 tablespoon olive oil
- 1 onion, diced
- 2 cloves garlic, minced
- 1 bell pepper, diced
- 1 zucchini, diced
- 1 cup sliced mushrooms
- 1 teaspoon dried oregano
- 1 teaspoon dried basil
- Salt and pepper to taste
- 1 can (15 ounces) diced tomatoes

- 2 cups baby spinach leaves
- Cooked whole grain pasta or brown rice for serving
- Grated Parmesan cheese for garnish (optional)

Instructions:

- Heat olive oil in a large skillet over medium heat. Add diced onion and minced garlic, and sauté until softened and fragrant, about 2-3 minutes.
- Add ground turkey to the skillet, breaking it up with a spoon, and cook until browned and cooked through.
- Add diced bell pepper, diced zucchini, sliced mushrooms, dried oregano, dried basil, salt, and pepper to the skillet. Cook for 5-7 minutes, or until the vegetables are tender.
- Stir in diced tomatoes (with their juices) and baby spinach leaves. Cook for an additional 2-3 minutes, until the spinach wilts and the mixture is heated through.
- Taste and adjust seasoning as needed.
- Serve the turkey and vegetable skillet over cooked whole grain pasta or brown rice.
- Garnish with grated Parmesan cheese, if desired.

- Enjoy this flavorful and nutritious dinner!

Health Benefits:

- Lean ground turkey is a good source of protein, which is essential for muscle repair and immune function.
- Vegetables such as bell peppers, zucchini, mushrooms, and spinach provide vitamins, minerals, and antioxidants, which can help reduce inflammation and support overall health.
- Whole grain pasta or brown rice offers complex carbohydrates and fiber, which can help stabilize blood sugar levels and support digestive health.

Preparation Time: Approximately 30 minutes.

8: Vegetable Lentil Soup

Ingredients:

- 1 tablespoon olive oil
- 1 onion, diced
- 2 carrots, diced
- 2 celery stalks, diced
- 2 cloves garlic, minced

- 1 teaspoon dried thyme
- 1 teaspoon dried rosemary
- 1 cup dried green or brown lentils, rinsed
- 6 cups vegetable broth
- 1 can (15 ounces) diced tomatoes
- 2 cups chopped kale or spinach leaves
- Salt and pepper to taste
- Fresh parsley for garnish (optional)

Instructions:

- Heat olive oil in a large pot over medium heat. Add diced onion, diced carrots, and diced celery. Sauté until softened, about 5 minutes.
- Add minced garlic, dried thyme, and dried rosemary to the pot. Cook for another 1-2 minutes, until fragrant.
- Add rinsed lentils, vegetable broth, and diced tomatoes (with their juices) to the pot. Bring to a boil, then reduce heat to low and simmer, covered, for 20-25 minutes, or until the lentils are tender.
- Stir in chopped kale or spinach leaves and cook for an additional 2-3 minutes, until wilted.

- Taste and adjust seasoning with salt and pepper as needed.
- Serve the vegetable lentil soup hot, garnished with fresh parsley if desired.
- Enjoy this comforting and nutritious dinner!

Health Benefits:

- Lentils are a good source of plant-based protein, fiber, vitamins, and minerals, which can help support digestion and provide sustained energy.
- Vegetables such as carrots, celery, kale, and spinach provide vitamins, minerals, and antioxidants, which can help reduce inflammation and support overall health.
- Herbs like thyme and rosemary add flavor and may have additional health benefits, including antioxidant and anti-inflammatory properties.

Preparation Time: Approximately 40 minutes.

9: Lemon Garlic Shrimp with Quinoa and Broccoli

Ingredients:

- 1 pound large shrimp, peeled and deveined
- 2 tablespoons olive oil
- 4 cloves garlic, minced
- Zest and juice of 1 lemon
- Salt and pepper to taste
- 1 cup quinoa, rinsed
- 2 cups vegetable broth or water
- 2 cups broccoli florets
- Fresh parsley for garnish (optional)

Instructions:

- In a large bowl, toss the shrimp with olive oil, minced garlic, lemon zest, lemon juice, salt, and pepper until evenly coated. Let marinate for 10-15 minutes.
- Meanwhile, in a saucepan, combine quinoa and vegetable broth or water. Bring to a boil, then reduce heat to low, cover, and simmer for 15-20 minutes, or until quinoa is cooked and liquid is absorbed.

- While the quinoa is cooking, steam or blanch the broccoli florets until tender-crisp. Drain and set aside.
- Heat a large skillet over medium-high heat. Add the marinated shrimp and cook for 2-3 minutes per side, or until pink and opaque.
- Once the quinoa is cooked, fluff it with a fork and divide it among serving plates.
- Arrange the cooked shrimp and steamed broccoli alongside the quinoa.
- Garnish with fresh parsley, if desired.
- Serve the lemon garlic shrimp with quinoa and broccoli hot.
- Enjoy this protein-rich and flavorful dinner!

Health Benefits:

- Shrimp is a lean source of protein, low in saturated fat, and rich in omega-3 fatty acids, which can help reduce inflammation and support heart health.
- Quinoa is a gluten-free whole grain rich in protein, fiber, vitamins, and minerals, which can help support digestion and provide sustained energy.

- Broccoli is packed with vitamins, minerals, and antioxidants, which can help reduce inflammation and support overall health.

Preparation Time: Approximately 30 minutes.

10: Mediterranean Stuffed Portobello Mushrooms

Ingredients:

- 4 large portobello mushrooms, stems removed
- 2 tablespoons olive oil
- 2 cloves garlic, minced
- 1/2 cup diced red bell pepper
- 1/2 cup diced zucchini
- 1/4 cup diced red onion
- 1/4 cup chopped fresh parsley
- 1/4 cup chopped Kalamata olives
- 1/4 cup crumbled feta cheese (optional)
- 1 teaspoon dried oregano
- Salt and pepper to taste
- Lemon wedges for serving

Instructions:

- Preheat the oven to 375°F (190°C). Line a baking sheet with parchment paper.
- Place the portobello mushrooms on the prepared baking sheet, gill side up.
- In a skillet, heat olive oil over medium heat. Add minced garlic and sauté until fragrant, about 1 minute.
- Add diced red bell pepper, diced zucchini, diced red onion, chopped fresh parsley, chopped Kalamata olives, dried oregano, salt, and pepper to the skillet. Cook for 5-7 minutes, or until the vegetables are tender.
- Spoon the vegetable mixture evenly into each portobello mushroom cap.
- If using, sprinkle crumbled feta cheese over the stuffed mushrooms.
- Bake in the preheated oven for 15-20 minutes, or until the mushrooms are tender and the filling is heated through.
- Remove from the oven and let cool slightly before serving.

- Serve the Mediterranean stuffed portobello mushrooms hot, with lemon wedges on the side for squeezing over the mushrooms.
- Enjoy this flavorful and satisfying dinner!

Health Benefits:

- Portobello mushrooms are low in calories and rich in vitamins, minerals, and antioxidants, which can help reduce inflammation and support overall health.
- Mediterranean-inspired vegetables such as bell peppers, zucchini, red onions, parsley, and olives provide vitamins, minerals, and antioxidants, which can help reduce inflammation and support heart health.
- Feta cheese offers protein and calcium, while also adding flavor to the dish (optional).

Preparation Time: Approximately 30 minutes.

Breast Cancer Snacks Recipes

1: Greek Yogurt Parfait

Ingredients:

- 1 cup plain Greek yogurt

- 1/2 cup mixed berries (such as strawberries, blueberries, raspberries)
- 1/4 cup granola
- 1 tablespoon honey or maple syrup (optional)
- Fresh mint leaves for garnish (optional)

Instructions:

- In a serving glass or bowl, layer plain Greek yogurt, mixed berries, and granola.
- Drizzle honey or maple syrup over the top, if desired.
- Garnish with fresh mint leaves for an extra burst of flavor and aroma.
- Serve immediately and enjoy this refreshing and nutritious snack!

Health Benefits:

- Greek yogurt is high in protein and probiotics, which can support digestive health and immune function.
- Berries are rich in antioxidants, vitamins, and fiber, which can help reduce inflammation and support overall health.

- Granola provides complex carbohydrates and fiber, offering sustained energy and promoting digestive health.

Preparation Time: Approximately 5 minutes.

2: Avocado Toast with Tomato and Basil

Ingredients:

- 2 slices whole grain bread, toasted
- 1 ripe avocado
- 1 small tomato, sliced
- Fresh basil leaves
- Salt and pepper to taste
- Red pepper flakes for garnish (optional)
- Lemon wedges for serving (optional)

Instructions:

- Halve the ripe avocado and remove the pit. Scoop out the flesh into a small bowl and mash it with a fork until smooth.
- Spread the mashed avocado evenly onto the toasted whole grain bread slices.
- Arrange tomato slices on top of the avocado spread.

- Tear fresh basil leaves and sprinkle them over the tomato slices.
- Season with salt and pepper to taste.
- If desired, garnish with red pepper flakes for a touch of heat.
- Serve the avocado toast with tomato and basil immediately, accompanied by lemon wedges for squeezing over the toast if desired.
- Enjoy this delicious and nutrient-packed snack!

Health Benefits:

- Avocado is rich in heart-healthy monounsaturated fats, vitamins, and minerals, which can help reduce inflammation and support overall health.
- Whole grain bread provides complex carbohydrates and fiber, offering sustained energy and promoting digestive health.
- Tomatoes are packed with vitamins, minerals, and antioxidants, which can help reduce inflammation and support immune function.

- Basil offers vitamins, minerals, and antioxidants, adding flavor and potential health benefits to the snack.

Preparation Time: Approximately 10 minutes.

3: Hummus and Veggie Platter

Ingredients:

- 1 cup hummus (store-bought or homemade)
- Assorted fresh vegetables for dipping (such as carrot sticks, cucumber slices, bell pepper strips, cherry tomatoes, snap peas)
- Whole grain crackers or pita bread, sliced (optional)

Instructions:

- Arrange the hummus in the center of a serving platter.
- Surround the hummus with assorted fresh vegetables for dipping.
- If desired, add whole grain crackers or sliced pita bread to the platter.
- Serve the hummus and veggie platter immediately, and enjoy dipping and snacking!

Health Benefits:

- Hummus is made from chickpeas (garbanzo beans), which are rich in protein, fiber, vitamins, and minerals, supporting digestive health and providing sustained energy.
- Fresh vegetables offer vitamins, minerals, and antioxidants, which can help reduce inflammation and support overall health.
- Whole grain crackers or pita bread provide complex carbohydrates and fiber, offering sustained energy and promoting digestive health.

Preparation Time: Approximately 10 minutes.

4: Almond Butter Apple Slices

Ingredients:

- 2 apples, cored and sliced
- 1/4 cup almond butter
- 2 tablespoons honey or maple syrup (optional)
- 2 tablespoons chopped almonds or walnuts (optional)
- Cinnamon for sprinkling (optional)

Instructions:

- Spread almond butter evenly onto the apple slices.
- Drizzle honey or maple syrup over the almond butter, if desired.
- Sprinkle chopped almonds or walnuts over the almond butter.
- For extra flavor, sprinkle cinnamon over the top.
- Serve the almond butter apple slices immediately, and enjoy this simple and nutritious snack!

Health Benefits:

- Almond butter is a source of healthy fats, protein, vitamins, and minerals, which can help reduce inflammation and support heart health.
- Apples provide vitamins, minerals, and antioxidants, which can help reduce inflammation and support digestive health.
- Honey or maple syrup adds natural sweetness, while chopped almonds or walnuts offer additional crunch and nutrients.

Preparation Time: Approximately 5 minutes.

5: Berry and Nut Yogurt Parfait

Ingredients:

- 1 cup plain Greek yogurt
- 1/2 cup mixed berries (such as strawberries, blueberries, raspberries)
- 2 tablespoons chopped nuts (such as almonds, walnuts, or pecans)
- 1 tablespoon honey or maple syrup (optional)
- 1/4 teaspoon vanilla extract (optional)

Instructions:

- In a serving glass or bowl, layer plain Greek yogurt, mixed berries, and chopped nuts.
- Drizzle honey or maple syrup over the top for sweetness, if desired.
- Optional: Stir in vanilla extract into the yogurt for extra flavor.
- Serve immediately and enjoy this delicious and nutritious snack!

Health Benefits:

- Greek yogurt is high in protein and probiotics, which can support digestive health and immune function.
- Berries are rich in antioxidants, vitamins, and fiber, which can help reduce inflammation and support overall health.
- Nuts provide healthy fats, protein, vitamins, and minerals, which can help reduce inflammation and support heart health.

Preparation Time: Approximately 5 minutes.

6: Veggie Sushi Rolls

Ingredients:

- 2 nori seaweed sheets
- 1/2 cup cooked quinoa
- 1/2 cucumber, julienned
- 1 carrot, julienned
- 1/2 avocado, sliced
- 2 tablespoons low-sodium soy sauce or tamari
- Pickled ginger and wasabi for serving (optional)

Instructions:

- Place a nori seaweed sheet on a clean surface, shiny side down.
- Spread cooked quinoa evenly over the nori sheet, leaving a 1-inch border at the top.
- Arrange cucumber, carrot, and avocado slices in a line along the bottom edge of the nori sheet.
- Starting from the bottom, tightly roll the nori sheet into a cylinder, using a bamboo sushi mat or your hands to help.
- Moisten the top border of the nori sheet with a bit of water to seal the roll.
- Repeat the process with the second nori sheet and remaining ingredients.
- Using a sharp knife, slice each sushi roll into bite-sized pieces.
- Serve the veggie sushi rolls with low-sodium soy sauce or tamari for dipping.
- Optional: Serve with pickled ginger and wasabi for extra flavor.

Health Benefits:

- Nori seaweed is rich in vitamins, minerals, and iodine, which can support thyroid health and provide essential nutrients.
- Quinoa is a gluten-free whole grain rich in protein, fiber, vitamins, and minerals, which can help support digestion and provide sustained energy.
- Vegetables such as cucumber, carrot, and avocado provide vitamins, minerals, and antioxidants, which can help reduce inflammation and support overall health.

Preparation Time: Approximately 20 minutes.

7: Edamame Hummus with Crudites

Ingredients:

- 1 cup shelled edamame (fresh or frozen)
- 2 tablespoons tahini
- 2 tablespoons lemon juice
- 1 clove garlic, minced
- 2 tablespoons olive oil
- Salt and pepper to taste

- Assorted raw vegetables for dipping (such as carrot sticks, cucumber slices, bell pepper strips)

Instructions:

- If using frozen edamame, cook according to package instructions. If using fresh edamame, steam until tender.
- In a food processor, combine the cooked edamame, tahini, lemon juice, minced garlic, olive oil, salt, and pepper.
- Blend until smooth, scraping down the sides of the food processor as needed.
- Taste and adjust seasoning if necessary.
- Transfer the edamame hummus to a serving bowl.
- Arrange the raw vegetables around the hummus for dipping.
- Serve immediately and enjoy this protein-rich and flavorful snack!

Health Benefits:

- Edamame is rich in plant-based protein, fiber, vitamins, and minerals, which can help support muscle repair, digestion, and overall health.

- Tahini provides healthy fats, protein, vitamins, and minerals, which can help reduce inflammation and support heart health.
- Raw vegetables offer vitamins, minerals, and antioxidants, which can help reduce inflammation and support immune function.

Preparation Time: Approximately 15 minutes.

8: Almond Butter and Banana Rice Cakes

Ingredients:

- 2 rice cakes
- 2 tablespoons almond butter
- 1 ripe banana, sliced
- 1 tablespoon chia seeds (optional)
- Drizzle of honey or maple syrup (optional)

Instructions:

- Spread almond butter evenly onto each rice cake.
- Arrange banana slices on top of the almond butter.
- Sprinkle chia seeds over the banana slices, if using.
- Optional: Drizzle honey or maple syrup over the top for added sweetness.

- Serve immediately and enjoy this quick and satisfying snack!

Health Benefits:

- Almond butter is a source of healthy fats, protein, vitamins, and minerals, which can help reduce inflammation and support heart health.
- Bananas provide vitamins, minerals, and carbohydrates, which can help replenish energy levels and support digestion.
- Rice cakes offer a gluten-free and low-calorie base for the snack, providing a crunchy texture without added fat or sugar.

Preparation Time: Approximately 5 minutes.

9: Cottage Cheese and Fruit Bowl

Ingredients:

- 1/2 cup low-fat cottage cheese
- 1/2 cup mixed fresh fruits (such as berries, sliced kiwi, pineapple chunks)
- 1 tablespoon chopped nuts (such as almonds, walnuts, or pecans)

- 1 teaspoon honey or maple syrup (optional)
- Dash of cinnamon (optional)

Instructions:

- In a bowl, scoop the low-fat cottage cheese.
- Arrange mixed fresh fruits on top of the cottage cheese.
- Sprinkle chopped nuts over the fruit and cottage cheese.
- Drizzle with honey or maple syrup for added sweetness, if desired.
- Optional: Sprinkle a dash of cinnamon over the top for extra flavor.
- Serve immediately and enjoy this protein-rich and refreshing snack!

Health Benefits:

- Cottage cheese is a good source of protein and calcium, which can help support muscle repair, bone health, and overall wellness.

- Mixed fresh fruits offer vitamins, minerals, and antioxidants, which can help reduce inflammation and support immune function.
- Nuts provide healthy fats, protein, vitamins, and minerals, which can help reduce inflammation and support heart health.

Preparation Time: Approximately 5 minutes.

10: Spinach and Feta Stuffed Mushrooms

Ingredients:

- 8 large mushrooms, stems removed
- 1 cup fresh spinach, chopped
- 1/4 cup crumbled feta cheese
- 2 tablespoons diced red bell pepper
- 1 clove garlic, minced
- 1 tablespoon olive oil
- Salt and pepper to taste

Instructions:

- Preheat the oven to 375°F (190°C). Line a baking sheet with parchment paper.

- In a skillet, heat olive oil over medium heat. Add minced garlic and diced red bell pepper, and sauté until softened, about 2-3 minutes.
- Add chopped fresh spinach to the skillet and cook until wilted, about 1-2 minutes.
- Remove the skillet from heat and stir in crumbled feta cheese. Season with salt and pepper to taste.
- Stuff each mushroom cap with the spinach and feta mixture.
- Place the stuffed mushrooms on the prepared baking sheet.
- Bake in the preheated oven for 15-20 minutes, or until the mushrooms are tender and the filling is heated through.
- Remove from the oven and let cool slightly before serving.
- Serve the spinach and feta stuffed mushrooms warm as a nutritious and savory snack!

Health Benefits:

- Mushrooms are low in calories and rich in vitamins, minerals, and antioxidants, which can help reduce inflammation and support overall health.
- Spinach is packed with vitamins, minerals, and antioxidants, which can help reduce inflammation and support immune function.
- Feta cheese offers protein and calcium, while also adding flavor to the snack.

Preparation Time: Approximately 25 minutes.

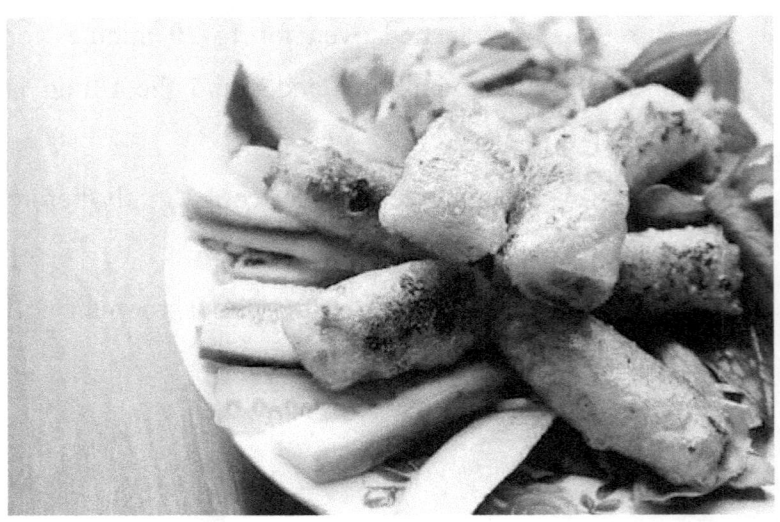

CONCLUSION

The Breast Cancer Cookbook stands not only as a collection of recipes but as a beacon of hope and support for those navigating the complexities of breast cancer.

Through its pages, individuals find not just nourishment for the body, but also empowerment for the spirit. Each recipe is crafted with care, blending the art of culinary expertise with the science of nutrition, tailored specifically to the unique needs of those affected by breast cancer.

Beyond its culinary offerings, this cookbook serves as a companion on the journey to wellness, offering guidance, encouragement, and a sense of community to its readers.

It fosters a deeper understanding of the role that nutrition plays in healing and resilience, empowering individuals to take charge of their health and well-being.

As we turn the final page, let us carry forward the lessons learned within these recipes—of strength, resilience, and the transformative power of nourishment. May this cookbook serve as a reminder that, even in the face of adversity, there is always a seat at the table for hope, healing, and the shared experience of breaking bread together.

www.ingramcontent.com/pod-product-compliance
Lightning Source LLC
Chambersburg PA
CBHW050323230526
45471CB00005B/2319